HOW TO FACE

LIFE'S BLACK HOLES

AND *OVERCOME*

HOW TO FACE
LIFE'S BLACK HOLES
AND *OVERCOME*

CM Harding

Arlene M. Harding

P & L Publishing
& Literary Services

ISBN: 9798396156463

Dedication

There are dangers that we face every day and many of them are bent on only one conclusion - to destroy us.

They will just continue to "Be There," waiting for an opportunity *to suck us into their space*!

This book is written with the hope of helping you AND ME to face those black holes, and overcome!

.

CONTENTS

Foreword

My first book – a thirty year project, entitled "<u>Commissioned by Gramma</u> <u>and Chosen by God</u>" – is now in the marketplace AND ALSO on Kindle-E Books. And according to the publishers, it is a success - they have given it five stars.

My Gramma would be proud to know the extent of her life's testimony.

Although for her, it all began many years ago while she was living with her daughter in Riviera Beach, Florida.

On a particular Sunday night she felt a heavy burden for the lost condition of her family and she began praying for them. They seemed to be headed, (and these are her words), "to hell in a handbasket". So, as she became very aware of her own mortality, she began asking God to raise-up someone to help her in this venture, to take the baton and carry it through to completion.

At the age of 98 trying to get some much needed rest amid the warm Florida temperatures, she drifted off into a deep sleep. Suddenly she awakened with a start, there was an" unusual, someone" in her room, standing by her bed.

He was dressed in a shining garment and carrying a sword in his right hand. She immediately determined that this must be an Angel.

He spoke to her these words that echoed through her

entire being, - "Izora, I have a message for you - WE have raised-up someone to take your place in interceding for your family's redemption!"

To her, it could mean only one thing, that She was about to depart this life. At her age, she was afraid to guess what that all entailed.

It is now sixty three years after that visitation, God has definitely kept His promise to bring into the ark of safety her family, at least that part that she had assumed the responsibility for.

There are only two members of her immediate family that are left to be brought in, and these are the toughest cookies of all. But with God all things are possible!

That promise, "With God all things are possible, to them that believe" is still being clung to by her helper, namely me.

So, with faith in my heart, I will continue to believe God, rather than to look at the circumstances.

I am retired now and am encouraged by the success of book number one. My publishers and editors have asked me to write another book along with a study guide, so here goes.

CM Harding

Introduction:
Bank Her to the Right, Now!

A few days back I was reading a story about the town of Victorville, California. It seems that Tumbleweeds are a common sight around the area. But in April 2019 that little town was inundated with those pesky thistle weeds.

The high winds of the Mojave Desert swept in so hard that these tumbleweeds almost took over the whole town.

No one expected the onslaught of these pesky critters, but here they were, and the only question now was, "how to deal with them."

Some reporter was heard to say, "such is life in the fast lane."

This story started me thinking, of our world and some of the strange things that's going on around us, and you have my word on it, there is more to come. This is just the tip of the iceberg.

In my mind I was taken aback to a windy cold Thursday in 1992. I was in a twin-engine Cessna at 10,000 feet above the gulf stream east of Florida.

The pilot and the owner, Marlin, seemed to be concentrating only on his stack of papers in his lap. He turned and pointed his pen at me and said, "she's all yours, my friend," and turned his attention back to his papers. Not another word was said for what seemed like an hour, but it was less than a minute. As he continued to fill out his custom declarations, I interrupted him with, "are- you-crazy- man?" I don't know how to fly a plane. Then he interrupted me with these immortal words, "It's just like driving a car."

I looked at him with consternation and said, "No sir, I have driven many different kinds of cars, but never have I flown an airplane, it's not the same."

But he insisted, "fly it or we will take a kamikaze dive into the ocean. Do you want that?" _So, I flew it_!

We were about half-way across the Caribbean heading for the Bahamas when right in front of us there appeared a massive bank of storm clouds that were awesome to look at.

I looked over at Marlin and asked, "And what do I do now?" he looked up from his paperwork and I could see the concern register on his face.

"See that dark-hole right in front of you he said, DO NOT, and I repeat, DO NOT go there, that thing will suck you into its center, where you will experience an electro-magnetic storm that will cripple this Cessna.

"What do I do, I asked. "Bank her to the right NOW, he said, what are you talking about", I asked - He just looked at me and went back to his paperwork, _so I banked her to the right_!

As I thought on this unusual situation, I began pondering the lesson that I learned there.

This was a, once- in-a-lifetime- experience for me. As I thought of this hair-raising experience, I began to formulate the thoughts for this that I am about to share with you. It is my hope that you will be aware as I am of the possibility _of "Black holes" popping up in your life's span._

1
The Black-Hole of Temptation

First let's determine what "A Black-Hole" is and what is it about those creatures that represents life itself.

A black hole is a region of space where the gravity pull is so strong that nothing can escape it. Not even electromagnetic particles of light can escape.

As I thought about this, I began to realize that black holes are a harbinger, a real sign of things to come, in life itself.

There are a lot of things that we must avoid, as we go through life.

Temptation is like a black hole.

Stay as far away from temptation as much as you can, for it can and will suck you into its existence and keep you from *your destination in life.*

I recall a story that I read many years ago.

As it goes, A huge battleship was plowing through the stormy seas in a foggy night, when the captain sees a light in the distance blinking a warning.

The captain immediately sent out a message that said, "Emergency! Collision inevitable! Change your course ten degrees to the south."

From the light in the distance came the reply, "emergency,

collision inevitable, change your course ten degrees to the north."

The captain gets a bit hot under the collar and sends back the same message, adding, "**I am the captain!**"

From the light came the answer, "Emergency, collision inevitable, change your course ten degrees to the north, <u>I am a third class seaman</u>." By this time the captain is furious, so he sends out what he believes to be the clincher, "Emergency, Emergency, collision inevitable. Change your course ten degrees to the south, "**I am a battleship!**"

Quickly the answer came back, "Emergency, collision inevitable, change your course ten degrees to the north, **I AM THE LIGHTHOUSE!**"

<u>So, at the insistence of the pilot of that Cessna, *I banked her to the right*</u> and went around that storm cloud, even though I thought, the pilot was out of his cotton-pickin'-mind, I just knew, that I knew, better.

This is so typical of life. It seems that there are always Black Holes, waiting in the balances, to suck us into *their darkness* and change your destination.

But you don't have to and let your life be changed by, "taking a short-cut" through, some "perceived- quick-access," just to get to where you think you ought to be.

There is an old song that was born in the fish markets of Nassau, and I think it tells it so well, *it goes like this*;

"*Never mind the noise of the market, just get the price of the fish.*"

So, let's cut to the chase.

In the experiences of life, there will always be Black Holes, waiting, with patience, for you to show up.

2
The Monster of Fear

Whether we are willing to admit it or not, FEAR is a black-hole, and it always shows up at a most inappropriate time, and at the most inconvenient places.

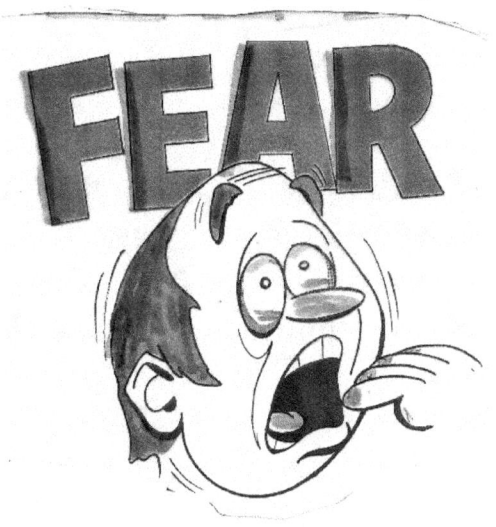

Most of us learn how to hide our fears as we grow older, but hide them, as we may, they still affect us and the quality of our lives.

The people that have studied the activities of the human brain have come up with some conclusions. *They state*:

The part of the brain that controls fear, is called "the Amygdala"- this is the area of the brain that becomes hyperactive and causes, what is known as "a Panic attack"- that area is known as, 'the fear center,' and it is what causes us to experience pain.

Dean Mobbs, of Caltech, division of Humanities and Social Sciences, reporting on the study done by his group, states; "when the defensive mechanisms malfunctions, it may result in an over exaggeration of "a perceived threat'. It causes an increase into the anxiety factor and then panic sets in".

This seems to be the tool that Satan endeavors to use in the lives of many Christians, to cause us, to make rash decisions. And if you fall for that trick, you are on your way into a Black-Hole and perhaps on your way to doing irreparable damage to yourself and even to those around you.

The downward spiral will continue to destroy the life and livelihood of many others, if the trend is continued.

So then, what do we do to stop, the entering-in-to, of this Black-Hole of fear?

Here are a few clues:
Number 1: Face your fears.
Name them - Are they real or not.

Call them out. Look at the evidence. What proof is there to corroborate them?

Now go back to the basics and ask yourself. "Is it possible for me to think clearly when I'm under the thumb of this real, or imaginary, perception"?

Keep in mind that "denial does not work," for fear is only as strong as you allow it to become.

Fear is a Nero-physiological response to a "perceived threat"- and it may only be *perceived*! Also keep in mind "The brave does not deny his fears, *but Triumph's over them.*"

Also try to remember that you are not alone. Even the animal kingdom must deal with this monster of fear.

The thing to do is, stand up with courage and conquer your fears.

Number two: Speak to your fears!
Don't blame someone else for the trauma you're facing.

The scripture says, "God has not given us a spirit of

bondage that we should always be afraid, but He has given us a spirit of love, power and a sound mind." And who do you know anyone that has Perfect Love, other than God?

So put the blame where it belongs,

As Jesus said, *"an enemy has done this"*!

Number three: Stand up with courage and wait with patience on the Lord to help you conquer your fears.

This is the only way to defeat these dragons that show up in your life.

Fear is a dragon and the only way to defeat it is, to kill it, before it kills you!

3
What Do I Do Next?

I remember the feelings that came over me as I took the controls of that Cessna…The hardest one to deal with was "the FEAR that I may crash this tin-can!"

And then I began to feel the panic of - "what do I do next."

Listen my friend, we were 10,000 feet above the ground, with nothing but space above, around and beneath us and that Cessna was loaded to the hilt. So one wrong move, on my part, and it would dive into the ocean at a tremendous rate of speed, and that ocean wasn't a very hospitable place if you were unprepared. And furthermore, I, who had no experience at all, _had the controls!_

I believe that I was almost to the place of being overcome to my fears and that was not a place that I wanted, or needed, to be!

And then what seemed like a good thought, came to me, "why not just put her on "Automatic-Pilot? -because my mind was doing, ten thousand flips a second, trying to come up with a solution.

What do I do? is there anything in my repertoire that could help me without ruining a special relationship with this man, who was giving me orders, and ignoring the fact that I had no experience to carry them out.

And then I remembered something that I read just a few days *ago;*

Author Claude Bristol, a Lawyer, a Lecturer, an investment banker and foreign correspondent and author of the best seller, TNT, The power within, *wrote,* There is dormant, in each individual, the faculty to succeed in whatever he desires, whatever the mind can conceive, the individual can achieve"!

But in my mind, there was not enough stored knowledge to use at such a time as this.

But according to Mr. Bristol there are two kinds of activities in the mind;

There is *"The Conscious Mind"*- and there is the *"SUB-conscious mind."*

The case-in-effect is "which area are we using at which time"?

The *sub-conscious mind* is an amazing mental library!

This was the secret of; *Henry Ford, Thomas Edison, Marconi the electric genius, Westinghouse, Andrew Carnegie, Albert Einstein and Charles Kettering*, they have all used what was written on the "Mental Library" of their Sub-conscious mind!

The SUB-conscious mind works like a magnet, to draw all the ingredients together effectively, so as to achieve your persistent picture!

Now here's the kicker:

Persistent FEAR...Doubt...Hate...-or- Happiness, Joy & Peace. Love, and wholeness - ALL can be brought-about by the mind, and telegraphed to the body, and as it reacts to this stimulus, it becomes as such.

The sub-conscious mind takes orders from the Conscious mind and can be amazingly creative AND, one surprising thing is, IT NEVER RESTS!

The Conscious mind sows the seed, *and* the Sub-conscious mind grows the plant!

The Sub-conscious mind has no power of choice! It only develops what is put into it. Like a computer does!

In other words, *We become what we THINK!*

In Proverbs 23:7 it says; "As a man thinks in his heart, so is he"!

"An idea or a purpose may be planted into the Sub-conscious mind by repetition of thought and empowered by faith and expectancy"!

Mr. Bristol says; "There is a "dominant" in each of us individuals- It is the faculty to succeed in whatever we put our mind to...What the mind can conceive, the individual can achieve"!

So, there are two areas of the mind:

Number 1 is, "The *Sub-conscious*" and *number 2* is, "The *Conscious.*"

Anything that Impresses you, is drawn like a picture on the canvas of your mind, and the Conscious mind, like a TV camera, is the receiver, and your enthusiasm is the transmitting power!

The Sub-conscious mind works like a magnet to draw all the ingredients together effectively so, as to achieve your persistent picture!

Persistent doubt, persistent hate, persistent fear, sickness, happiness, joy, peace, and love, ALL can be brought-about by the mind and telegraphed to the body- AND EVERY PART WILL REACT TO THIS STIMULI!

The Sub-conscious mind takes orders from the Conscious mind and is amazingly creative, It never rests!

The *Conscious mind* plants the seed and the *sub-conscious* grows the plant!

But the sub-conscious has no power of choice. It only develops what is put-into it, something like a computer... So it is with us we become what we think!

Proverbs 23:7 says, *"As a man thinks in his heart, so is he"*!

Now to bring this plane in for a landing;

An idea or a purpose *may be planted in the sub-conscious* mind BY repetition of thought AND empowered by faith and expectancy…And if we truly believe that God is All-mighty and all-powerful, and that we can do all things thru Him- Then we would think on these things and convince ourselves of them by confession of such!

For example, Hitler practiced the destruction of, not only the Jews but all of mankind, But first he started thinking it and then he believed it and he stated the lie long enough and LOUD enough coercing most people to believe it *and then act upon it*!

A man had an auto accident with no apparent injuries, but he continues to feel a slight twinge in his head because he believes that he was injured there!

A man went to a Guru for some help and advice. He is told that he has heart trouble. He dies of a heart attack because he believed the guru!

A lady continues to testify that for most of her youth she has been in bondage, over what, she does not know, but her whole life is messed-up. She says, "I know I need to have victory over these things, but there seems to be a communication gap between her mind and her heart."?!

There needs to be a determination made *between what is* and what is not. The mind needs to be renewed by a greater power than the mind itself, and that GREATER POWER is where the Holy Spirit comes into the picture.

Paul says in Philippians 2:5 "let this mind be in you as was in Christ Jesus"!

We should pray this way till the answer comes, "Lord give me control of my mind as of this moment *and we should believe in our hearts that it is so*"!

If you are truly convinced that God is All Mighty, and All powerful, and that we can do all things thru Him- Then we would think of these things and convince ourselves of them, by confession that these things are so!

And avoiding the black holes in our lives, we need to begin at the beginning with Paul's advice, "Let this mind be in you as was in Christ Jesus."

And Romans 12:1-2 says, "I beseech you therefore, brethren, by the mercies of God, that ye present your bodies a living sacrifice, holy, acceptable unto God, which is your reasonable service."

And be not conformed to this world: but be ye transformed by the "renewing of your mind", that ye may prove what is that good, and acceptable, and perfect, will of God.

One of the most deceptive things that black holes bring about into our lives is indecision.

Indecision hastens things! and causes panic. In that state, everything calls loudly *for a decision, good or bad. All it wants is a decision*—No time for thinking, praying, or planning. Just hurry-up and "make a decision. *A decision must be made NOW!"*

Figure out what God wants later. Who cares what the family needs. You are here, in the middle of no-where and they are probably off somewhere shopping. So it's decision time and NOW!

And in the approach of that black hole, you had better take thirty deep breaths and try to squelch that thing -or- you are headed for DESTRUCTION!

In the flight across the Caribbean there was one thing that I did not want to do - and that was, to be late getting to my destination. Because, on the Island where we were headed, when it gets dark, it gets dark! Darker than anything you have ever imagined. There are no streetlights, unless a generator is running. And when the generator is shut down, which happens every night about bedtime, it becomes pitch black, the mosquitoes (which are like little demons,) begin their blood sucking ways.

So, I wanted to get to that landing strip quickly- in order to get to the next location where I would be spending the night- before the lights went out.

But Marlin said, "Bank her to the right and go all the way around the storm clouds."

Mt response was, "Brother, we are losing precious time, what will that do to our schedule?"

"Bank her right" was all he said, *so to the right we went*! I had to muster all my faculties and do what the pilot said, for once again I thought I knew that he was wrong, simply because I felt, *that I knew, better than he did.*

4
PANIC: A Perceived Danger

Many years ago, I was the chef on board an amazingly large passenger ship.

That was a special time in my teenage life to be in-charge of the galley which was an awesome responsibility.

I happened one stormy night as we were crossing the gulf stream off of Florida, that a massive storm arose, and it almost swamped the ship. The dining room doors broke loose from their latches and water was filling up the dining room. It just happened to be my responsibility to get out of bed and secure the doors, which was no small task.

As I worked my way around the drop-leaf dining room table, half of it flew up and when it came back down my left shinbone was in the way, though the bruise was painful, I didn't have time to pay any attention to the burning sensation I felt at that moment.

The dining room was secured, and I went back to bed. But upon waking up at four O'clock am, to start preparing for the breakfast, it was then that I realized that I had a problem. My leg was swollen so badly that my pant leg was torn up to my thigh and I was unable to walk on that leg.

It was my good fortune that we were in port in Nassau, Bahamas, so the captain gave me transportation to the company doctor. I spent thirty days under the care of the doctor before I could return to the ship.

One of the things that caused me almost to panic was "will I be able to go back to my job and maintain my position as the head chef of that huge outfit"? with over a hundred crewmembers plus the tremendous number of passengers. One thing was for sure, my lifestyle was about to be changed.

I am not sure how it started but Panic was creeping into my space.

Here is where the third black hole. And maybe the most insidious of all begins, it is the black-Hole of Panic, and this one is a killer!

Panic produces a sudden intense fear, that triggers a fever-like physical reaction to warn you that there is imminent danger. In reality, there may not be any danger at all. But it's a very frightening thing!

It also makes you feel 'out of control', like you are about to have a heart attack, or even about to die.

I was talking with one of my doctors who told me that he had been given the Covid-9 Vaccine AND had a reaction to the medicine. He spent the next three nights with sweating, chills, trembling, very restricted breathing, weakness, and dizziness, also tingling in the hands, chest pains and nausea.

This is exactly what happens when panic takes over. And to top it off, the Adrenal Gland begins to pump more Adrenaline into the blood stream. The muscles become heightened and breathing becomes laborious. As a result, you need more Oxygen, and even your sugar begins to spike. In other words, this thing can reap havoc in your life!

Unless you take back control of your life immediately, it will continue to pop up, and at the most inconvenient of times.

It is suggested that you can make friends with your adrenaline but be quick about it, and be firm, with it!

Some have found that a quick shower in cold water, for 30 minutes, and then adjust to hot water, for the same amount of time, seems to work. The only problem with this solution is, you are not always in a location to follow this scenario.

These attacks do not come at a time of your convenience. Their "soul-crushing" visits and the phobia associated with them, can cause you to become socially withdrawn and out of control, which can lead to depression.

There are numerous medications that are available to help, such as beta blockers and others. But unless you take control, of this monster, you will find the cure is almost as bad as the disease. Because if continued over a long period, this can lead to a chemical dependency and instead of a cure. It enhances the power of the problem. This can suck you into its black hole of panic and the dangers are myriad.

Lack of self-esteem and productivity can be, only a few of the dangers, you will have to deal with.

Fear of panic attacks can become the central focus of your life and as a result you will have to live with the overwhelming prospect of what is known as, panic-disorder.

Try to develop a list of what is known as, "adrenaline rush" activities, such as social interaction, a commitment to things that will improve your life. These will depend on your lifestyle and your preferences of activities.

You may have to develop your own personal list of activities that are suited to your way of life.

You may have, "a Caribbean soul, that you can hardly control," but most people don't. So the development of lists is up to you!

What If, all that you have been going through was, just "a perception"? What if, an enemy has crept-in and sowed these seeds of deception, in your garden overnight, and you are allowing them to grow into full blown weeds of fear and depression. What if, you are the only one who can pull these weeds out and give yourself a fruitful garden?!

Remember, your past does not determine your future. YOU make that determination!

It is well documented that many well-meaning individuals, have been sucked into the grip of this black hole of panic, and because of its fear, have been overcome by a monster known as depression.

One of the biggest monsters in my life, as a child, was the fear of heights. Whenever I got higher than twenty feet above the ground, I began to feel panic begin to creep in.

After I became an adult, I decided I would conquer that fear. So early one morning I got into my car, drove to Jupiter, Florida and took the challenge. I climbed to the top of the lighthouse, which had over one hundred steps, and the process, to defeating that monster, began.

This was quite a daring challenge for me because I was still in the early stages of recovery from open heart surgery.

But climb, I did, with one goal in mind, and that was to conquer my fears of heights.

As I stood at the top of that lighthouse, overlooking the beautiful gulf-stream-waters, it was at that point that I realized this might not have been a good idea! As I looked down to the ground, dizziness began creeping into my space and I almost panicked.

But I felt that this was only a "perceived danger," and so I decided to stay and take control of my situation, to understand it, cope with it, and it was at that point that I mastered my fears!

My only danger, at that point, was from walking back down those hundred plus steps. But thank God, my whole perception had changed, for I had conquered that dragon of fear.

The Apostle Paul gave us this advice in, 2nd Timothy1:7, "God has not given us a spirit of bondage to fear, but a spirit of love, power and a sound mind."

And with that "God given soundness of mind" we can master all our fears.

Jesus said in John14:1 "Do not let your heart be troubled" in other words "don't be afraid."

In Isaiah 41:10-11 it says; "Fear Not for I AM is with you, be not dismayed, for I AM your God; I will strengthen you, I will help you; I will uphold you with the Right-Hand of My Righteousness."

King David said in Psalm 27:1, "The Lord is my light and my Salvation; whom shall, I fear? The Lord is the strength of my life, of whom shall I be afraid?"

David also said, "What time I am afraid, I will trust in the Lord." But the Prophet Isaiah puts it more succinctly, sort of, in plain clothes, he said "I will trust and NOT be afraid,"

To bring it all home, when Jesus went into the Synagogue in His hometown of Nazareth, He stood up and read from the book of Isaiah. Which He opened to Isaiah 61:1--- (see Luke 4:18-), and He read, "The Spirit of the Lord is on me, because he has anointed me to proclaim good news to the poor. He has sent me to proclaim freedom for the prisoners, the recovery of sight for the blind, to set the oppressed free, to proclaim the year of the Lord's favor."

This scripture points us to God's plan and if followed, it will keep us from the black holes that seek to invade our space daily. The only way to avoid these menaces is to turn to Jesus Christ and rely fully on Him!

Now ponder this; - A quote from a message that I heard:

There seems to be a "A loss of compass" (or at least a broken one) in today's world. There is no such thing as "An American Angel" to keep us from hurting and being the target of someone else's perversion. God Loves THE WHOLE WORLD and he loves you too!

Remember there have been those who have given so much for so many and yet they seemed NOT to have been rewarded in this life.

They have been left behind in the shadows. Fear stalked them and they were left alone to panic under the weight of life. But you need not fear for, their victory is yours as well. So keep-on-keeping-on till the storm passes over!

5
Breeders of: The Lack of Hope

"Black holes" are a well-known commodity when it comes to losing hope.

One of the most crucial times in American history was the year 2020, and the introduction of, the ungodly virus, known as Covid-19. This was, and still is, a time of fear and panic for many. The reason is, lack of hope. Saturated by many reports of, the totals affected, the deaths, which seems to be into the millions, that came about as a result of being infected, many have gotten on a downward slope without any reason to hope.

Many of our friends and family have contracted this virus and some have even died from the effects of its constricting and rigorist results.

Those mask's that seemed to work, most of the time are now being questioned as a 'reason for' the spread of a new strain called, "the African-version" of Covid-19.

In this invasion, we have experienced a tremendous loss of hope.

Businesses have been closed, sports have been curtailed, schools have been canceled and the Church has even been affected.

Recently the worship team, at the church where we attend, shared a song with these words "I raise A Hallelujah, in the presence of my enemies, I will continue till fear is defeated, and up from the ashes HOPE will arise, So I'll Raise A Hallelujah"!

We are amid "a pandemic that is destroying our hope," And as a reporter on CBS News, speaking of the vaccinations, said, "The Vaccine is more of an Inoculation for hope" rather than a cure for a virus.

America and all the world needs something, or someone, to give us some hope.

The Prophet Jeremiah in the book of Lamentations 3:18-24, in his distress commiserates, "I said, my strength and my hope is gone, and all I can remember is my misery is, bitterness and grief have overcome me, BUT then, I thought of the Lord's Mercy as the only reason I am not consumed, for His mercy and compassion is new every morning, Great is Thy faithfulness, O' God, for now I have hope, You are my portion and there is hope in You O' Lord."

The old song, "On Christ the solid rock I stand, all other ground is sinking sand," gives us hope. *It continues*, "My hope is built on nothing less than Jesus' blood and righteousness." And like the old prophet, when we remember that "God always keeps His promises, *we have a reason for hope*!

Just one more old song, that is appropriate here, the title is "*I am free*, "I am free from the fear of tomorrow, I am free from the guilt of my past, I have traded my shackles for a glorious song, I am free, praise the Lord, free at last."

Now there's a word for you, Free from the guilt of my past!

Whether it is from the past or the present, guilt is a destructive commodity!

As a counsellor, I have heard many stories of regret; "A child has gone wrong," the hope that the parents had for that son or daughter has become a means of depression, Mom and

Dad now blame themselves for the decisions of a prodigal son or daughter. Who have made their own decisions. For some unknown reason, the parents are now allowing the guilt for it to make a mess of THEIR lives. Their relationship with each other is now in danger of falling apart.

Guilt can be just as dangerous as fear and can put a strangle-hold on hope, if allowed to continue.

But no amount of guilt can change the past, just as no amount of worry can help the future.

Here's a quote from missionary Tom Benegas, who almost lost his wife to Covid.

"Worry is a non-existent entity. It brings anxiety, and anxiety brings fear, and fear brings depression," so what are we to do? We should meditate upon the Word of God and thru IT, we will be given the answer, FAITH WINS!" And don't forget to pray!

6

The Blame Game

The fourth thing that Black holes are famous for is "Blaming someone, anyone, even God, _for our troubles._"

Most people are acquainted with a man called JOB, though, maybe, not with the extent of his troubles.

He lost his children, his cattle, his sheep and along with all of that, his wife, and his health. Job's friends and even his wife, counseled him to, "Curse God and die," in other words, Blame God for all your troubles!

But Job knew that God was his only hope of deliverance. So to blame God would circumvent the process for his future recovery. Remember, there will always be someone waiting in the balances to pour out "their version of guilt," that you are supposed bear and take the responsibility for, even suffer the pain for it all.

Dr. Richard Dobbins, the founder of Emerge Ministries, _used to make a statement that I will always remember,_ "The quality of your mind reflects the value of your choices. So don't let someone else determine what decisions you make, what you think, and the choices you make."

There are those who are like the story of the two skunks heading south out of Georgia, looking for a warmer climate in Florida.

When they came in the vicinity of Jacksonville, where

there is a large papermill operating, on skunk said to the other, "Phew, what's that I smell, I've gotta' have some of that." Now everyone is aware that papermills tend to stink-up the whole are, around where they are, and this one was no different.

And one thing about skunks, they love stink!

The other skunk answered his comrade, "it must be a dragon because it is puffing-out smoke, let's go and see so we can avail ourselves of some of, whatever that is."

That is what is known as "Stinkin'-thinkin'!"

And that's exactly what is in store for those who let their choices be determined by others.

Someone coined the phrase, "Others may, you may not!"

TD Jakes said, "Your choices *are your gods*! but your mind-set is, *who you really are!*"

Don't let your feelings lead you into a mis-guided relationship, the best thing to do is, let your views coincide with what God says and make your decisions based on what He directs.

The Apostle Paul has a lot to say about this in Romans 8:..

He says; "The person who is led by the *flesh* is hostile toward God because he will not subject himself to the law of God, really he is not able to." (7) This kind of person is a slave to sin, and he is incapable of doing the things that a believer should.

Paul's view of "life in Christ" is this; It is empowered by the Spirit of God and then he goes on to describe the difference between the flesh and the Spirit, in the 5th chapter of Galatians, here he urges us to "Walk in the Spirit so that we would not fulfill the lust of the flesh", Paul indicates that there is an internal struggle going on between our flesh and the Spirit. And then he gives us the outcome of listening to the flesh and the blessing of obeying the Spirit.

In Galatians 5:19-26 Paul says, "*The acts of the flesh* are obvious: they are, sexual immorality, impurity, and debauchery; idolatry and witchcraft; hatred, discord, jealousy, fits of rage, selfish ambition, dissensions, factions and envy; drunkenness, orgies, and the like. I warn you, as I did before, that those who live like this will not inherit the kingdom of God.

But the fruit of the Spirit is love, joy, peace, forbearance, kindness, goodness, faithfulness, gentleness and self-control. Against such things there is no law. Those who belong to Christ Jesus have crucified the flesh with its passions and desires. Since we live by the Spirit, let us keep in step with the Spirit. Let us not become conceited, provoking, and envying each other. (6:7-10) do not be deceived: God cannot be mocked. A man reaps what he sows. Whoever sows to please their flesh, from the flesh will reap destruction; whoever sows to please the Spirit, from the Spirit will reap eternal life. not give up. [10] Therefore, as we have opportunity, let us do good to all people, especially to those who belong to the family of believers.

Now less I leave you with that horrific list and you say, how in the world are we supposed to make it through?

He declares boldly, "If we live in the Spirit, let us also WALK in the Spirit."

If we live according to our fleshly desires, we will reap the result of what the flesh gives!

But if we live according to the dictates and leadings of The Spirit, we will reap the results, 'Life Everlasting', which is, an immortal, Abiding, Endless, Infinite, Deathless-never-ending, unbroken, un-interrupted, unique and without equal, in other words "Life without end", that's what awaits those who 'Live by the Spirit of God!"

And then Paul goes on to say in Romans 8:1-2, "There is therefore now, no condemnation for those who are in Christ Jesus, because through Christ Jesus and the law of the Spirit, who gives life, we are set us free from the law of sin and death."

7
Mountain Dreamers

One day while at work for Southeastern University, I was driving down El Prado, the main street of the campus. It was a dreary day because we were having a tropical downpour.

It was then that I noticed a piece of paper lying on a bench, that the rain had almost soaked into a soggy pile of pulp.

For some unknown reason, I felt, for some reason, an urge to stop and rescue that paper, it might be that some student had forgotten it and left it there but would need it later.

So, I stopped, picked it up, dried it off and put it in the glove compartment of my golf cart.

Several days later it was still there, so I decided to check out this important and unusual piece of paper.

It was something called "The mountain dreamer."

As I examined it, I was motivated to read on; This is the content:

"It doesn't interest me what you do for a living, I want to know what you ache for and if you dare dream of meeting your heart's longing.

It doesn't interest me how old you are, I want to know if you will risk looking like a fool for love, for your dream, for the adventure of being alive.

It doesn't interest me what planets are squaring your moon.

I want to know if you have touched the center of your own

sorrow, or if you have been opened to life's betrayals or have become shriveled and closed from fear of further pain.

I want to know if you can sit with pain, mine or yours, without moving to hide it or to fade it, or trying to fix it.

I want to know if you can be with Joy, mine or yours, and if you can dance in your wilderness and let ecstasy fill you to the tips of your toes, without cautioning yourself to be careful, to be realistic, to remember the limitations of being human.

It doesn't interest me if the story you're telling me is true.

All I want to know is, can you disappoint another to be true to yourself; or can you bear the accusation of betrayal and not betray your own soul, if you can be faithless and therefore still trustworthy.

I want to know if you can see beauty even when it's not pretty, every day, and if you can source your own life from its presence.

I want to know if you can live with failure, yours and mine, and still stand on the edge of the lake and shout to a silver moon, "YES!"

It doesn't interest me to know where you live or how much money you have. I want to know if you can get up, after a night of grief and despair, weary and bruised to the bone, and do what needs to be done to feed the children.

It doesn't matter to me who you know or how you came to be where you are. *I want to know if you will stand in the center of the fire with me and not shrink back.*

It doesn't matter to me where or what or with whom you studied.

I want to know what sustains you, from inside, when all else falls apart!

I want to know if you can be alone with yourself and if you truly, like the company you keep, in the empty moments of life."

That was a very revealing find and as I turned the page over I noticed something else interesting. it also included some interesting facts concerning *"Cognitive Decline". known as MCI (Mild-Cognitive-Impairment).*

"What seems to be, many times, like Dementia and Alzheimer, may be just a slow decline caused by aging. Concerns by family members over miss-placed keys or forgetting where glasses were left; many times, are because of familiarity.

Much of the diagnosis's are because of these concerns.

It has been found that 46% of those diagnosed were able to return to a normal lifestyle, functioning normal.

Many of the concerns were because of health issues, including stress, and had improved within six months.

Many were able to return to work and normal activities. This paper was worth the stop even in the rain.

This was quite a find, and so I include it here to enhance the contents of these things I'm writing about."

8
The Trap: Excuses

"Black holes" it seems, are the cause for many of the strange things that happen to us, *things that most of the time, could've been avoided*. But carelessly, we go on our merry way, blaming others, circumstances, and even God, for all our problems?

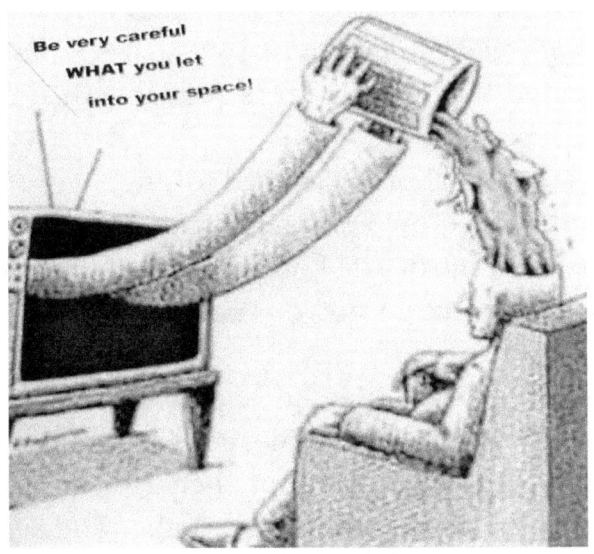

Remember; Adam blamed Eve. Eve blamed the serpent. Cain blamed Abel's choice of offerings. But God did not accept any of their excuses!

There's a song called "Excuses" that *the Kings Men* used to sing that really brings this into view;

"Excuses, excuses, you hear them every day, the devil will supply them if from church you stay away. When people come to know The Lord, the devil always loses, so to keep these folks away from church, he offers them excuses!"

In the summer it's too hot, in the winter it's too cold, in the springtime the weather is just right and there's lots of places to go. It's up to the mountains, down to the beach, or we'll just stay at home with the family. The sermons are to long, or maybe they're to short, The preacher ought to preach with d-i-g-n-i-t-y, instead of stomp and snort." Excuses, excuses. The devil knows how to supply an excuse for every situation, and if you listen to him, he will lead you smack-dab into a Black-Hole!

According to Marlin, *"If you're sucked into one of those Critters, you will need to have a greater power than any twin engine can supply, if you hope to get out.*

Thank God that this power is available thru the Name of Jesus!

There is an old chorus we used to sing;

"We've got the power, in the Name of Jesus, we've got the power, in the Name of The Lord. Though Satan rages, we will not be defeated, we've got the power, in the Name of the Lord."!

That's what Jesus tried to show His disciples in Luke 10:18-19. He replied to their questions with, "I saw Satan fall like lightning from heaven. But then He said, now, I have given you authority to trample on snakes and scorpions and "over all the power of the enemy", and nothing shall be any means hurt you".

If you will take the Word of Jesus for it, you will live in freedom!

9
Stressed-Out

The thing that stands-out as a Black Hole, and is waiting in line for you to take a trip with it, is called "S-T-R-E-S-S!"

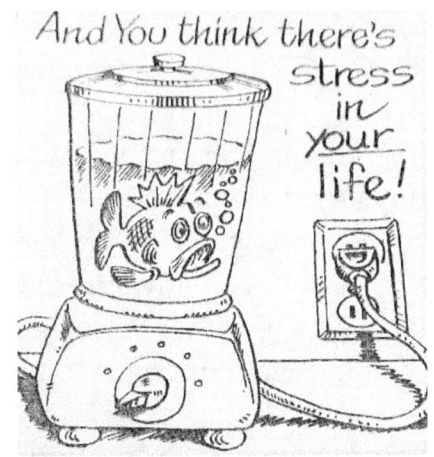

And You think there's stress in your life!

I remember reading about a close friend of mine who dedicated his life to the work of God and was serving as a Missionary.

I just knew that, if anyone would live till he was 99, and still be in good health, it was Jim!

We played touch football together when we were together in college, one time on the field of play he and I got tangled-up in an "I have-it-*because*-I-touched-you- first" situation, which caused both of us to fall and roll over and over hanging-on to that pig-skin, I came out of the roll all skinned up and bruised in places that I didn't know I had places.

But Jim was clean enough that he could go right back into class with no trouble at all.

After many years on the mission field this couple came home for a little rest and relaxation, and as usual, there was the preverbal medical check-up required before getting into the home phase of their lives, which was the fund raising and hopefully a little rest and relaxation. The doctors gave Jim a glowing report, everything was good, all his vitals were on target and the heart was in good condition.

After the long day at the doctor's office, Jim came home and gave his wife the glowing report. She rejoiced with him and went back into the kitchen to continue to fix supper, while Jim sat on the couch and relaxed with the joy of knowing, all-is-well!

While in the kitchen his wife, though happy for the glowing report, began to feel uneasy about something and returned to say something to Jim. He was stretched out on the couch fast asleep, so she went back to the kitchen to continue her cooking.

But still feeling uneasy about something she returned to check on her husband. After a third time checking and still having this strange feeling, she went over to where he lay and checked his pulse, he was laying there so unusually still, she checked his pulse once again, but there was none. To her amazement he was dead. The heart that was supposed to be so strong, had given out.

After calling the paramedics and having them examine him, the doctors said he suffered a massive heart attack.

While talking with the doctor, she was surprised to hear him say, "the ol' stress-factor" is to blame.

Stress is a silent killer! It causes the heart to be over - taxed and to suddenly stop.

Stress will also causes you to make a lot of mistakes and not realize it until much later.

How many times have we asked ourselves, *Why did I make such a stupid statement? Why did I act so out of character just now?*

At one point in my life, I used to be a perfectionist. There was "a place for everything, and everything was supposed to be in its place" and if it wasn't, I would become, for lack of a better word, stressed-out!

Stress is a Black-hole that will pull everyone into its confines sooner-or-later.

Stress will cause you to wake up from a sound sleep with sweat pouring down from your brow, wondering what's going on?!

And stress won't let you get back to sleep for hours. *How many times have I had to rebuke that spirit over and over 'til finally sleep came?*

There is a story that I remember reading of a Pastor who went to his doctor one afternoon, he was concerned because he was having all the symptoms of a heart attack.

The doctor treated him for several months, with the same symptoms every time, and he seemed to be getting no better. He tried several new remedies, and still nothing was working.

So the doctor tried some counseling, to try to circumvent the problem.

Pastor, he said, "Do you believe God's Word"?

"Of course, I do" replied the pastor, "I'm a preacher of the Word of God, sir, and I believe all that book"!

"But, do you believe <u>ALL the Word</u>"? Asked the doctor again?

"Hey doc, why all the strange questions" asked the pastor? Well, the doctor replied, "If, as you say, you believe all the Word of God, then what about the Verse that say's "I AM the Lord that healeth thee"?

There was a strange silence for a while and then the Pastor spoke very slowly and very distinctly, "I guess so, sir", he said, "I have some repenting to do. So if you'll please leave the room, I'll have a little talk with Jesus"!

About fifteen minutes or so, the doctor returned and found the Pastor sitting, very quiet and serene, "Is everything ok", asked the doctor, *"Yes" replied the Pastor,* with a big smile on his face, "How much do I owe you doctor", asked the Pastor, "Nothing" replied the doctor. Now I know you believe the Word you preach."

Stress does not have to have *a particular type of person to suck into its Black Hole;* it will take all kinds, including you and me!

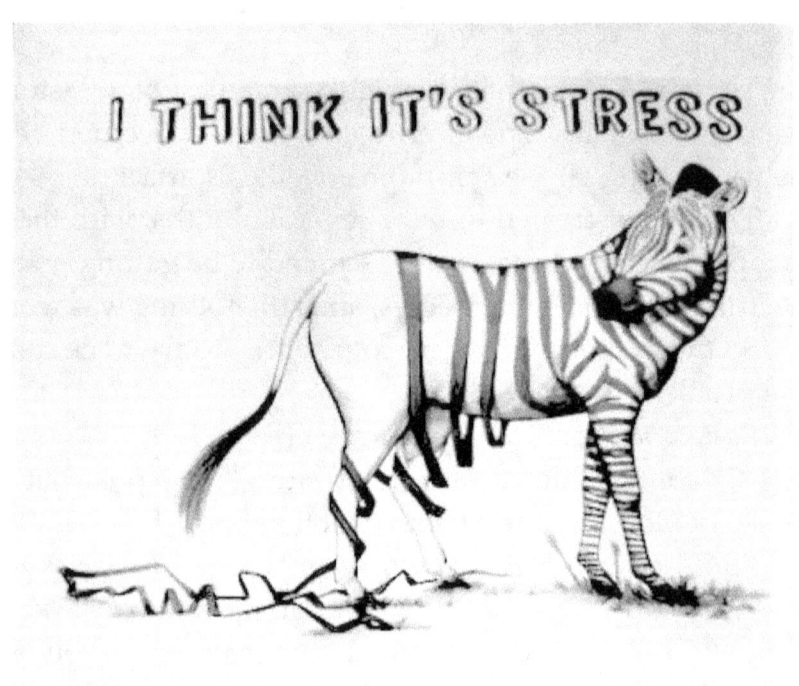

10
In the Know, Brother

The Black Hole that seeks to suck you in is, "wanting to know what's going to happen, before it happens".

I read the other day of the perfect solution for anyone with this type of mentality. *Your need is to "Trust-in-The-Lord with-all-your-heart-and not to lean on your own understanding," or on anyone else's understanding*!

Now, if you are one of those, King Saul type, who relies on, what is known today as, "psychic services," please remember, your answers that you get, will be coming from " The Father of Lies," Satan!

This service is popular among the most unassuming classes of people, *businessmen and women, the rich, the well-educated, it transcends all races, creeds, and ages, even financial status*. They are all wanting to know the future.

As a result of this curiosity, there has come into being a new business called "Psychic Services" one of the fastest growing businesses in the USA. It employs almost 100 thousand people who are primarily mediums, astrologers, palm readers, and fortune tellers. It generates over 2 billion dollars in revenue a year.

King Saul got caught-up in this farce during his reign as King of Israel. He wanted to know how his battles would turn out before they came into being. And he couldn't wait on the old Prophet Samuel, to hear from God. So he turned to a medium for the answers. The only problem for him was, after getting the wrong advice, he committed *suicide!*

When you leave God out of the equations and try to find another way to understand the future, your life is in danger!

Psychics do not know the future!

These fortune-tellers-tools, they are manufactured guesses.

When looking at their success or lack of the same, Benjamin Bradford says; "*They failed* in predicting the 911 disaster. *They failed* to predict the tsunami in Japan that destroyed so many people. *They failed* to predict the global economic collapse and so many other things. So why would anyone want to trust these crackpots? Just imagine how many lives could've been saved had they given us warnings of all these disasters".

But they didn't, because they are just fakers. They have nothing to give and that's what you get, *nothing!*

Just another Black Hole to suck as many as possible into their financial gains department.

Listen-up. Here's a great quote from David Levy (media consultant of the Friends of Israel magazine). "God alone, knows the end from the beginning and He not only foretells the future, He determines it!"

So if you want to know what's coming-up, you don't need "psychic's services," you need to Go to the source, God's Word! Bible prophecy, is simply "History written in advance!"

11
Stubbornness!

NOW to The Black Hole of stubbornness.

The world's number one "Stubborn candidate" WAS the Pharaoh of Egypt!

He lost his life because of his stubbornness!

You see he had a dogged determination to "not change his attitude" no matter what Moses or even God said!

The error for Pharaoh was that of refusing to admit that he was wrong. He was a Bullheaded man!

The BIG question is, *are we as Americans* making the same mistake today? Are we projecting ourselves as the most powerful and prosperous nation in the world, and even God should be pleased to have us around, No matter what we do, He should still be glad the He has us to lean-on!?

But with a national media, that's gone crazy, and a political system that looks more like Rome, back in the days of Jesus, *we seem to be headed back to the Egyptian curse, of Pharaoh.*

Is Pharaoh still alive today, OR can anyone identify who's behind all the crazies going on?

We are experiencing a "miniature" of what must've gone on, *when Lucifer rebelled against God and tried to take over the rule of heaven.*

Rest assured, Lucifer is back at it again, he's trying to take full control of the only nation on earth that has been, for over two hundred years, a bastion of freedom for the world to see, just a little of what God's Kingdom will be like.

Satan cannot stand the thought of peace and safety for all, when his idea for mankind, is hate and destruction.

Let's go back again into Pharaoh, back in his hay-day.

When He found, living right in his backyard, what a find it was, he proceeded to make slaves of them and he even prospered for a while. But the God of Heaven showed up. The one he forgot about because he had all the gods that he needed, or so he thought. And with all his gods, he had the feeling that nothing could go wrong, but he was wrong!

Egypt had a god for every occasion, and every evil purpose. One could conjure-up, crocodile gods, cat gods, frog gods, Isis, Osiris, Horus, Amun, Ra, Hathor, Bastet, Thoth, Anubis, Ptah, and many more (2,000) greater or lesser gods.

So, Pharaoh thought he had all his bases covered and that his gods could protect him under any circumstances, but again, he was wrong.

Because, the God of heaven, who is the God of power and wisdom and knowledge, the one who is the FIRST and the LAST, the beginning and the end, creator God, showed up, and took control of the situation.

And be it known, to all, that this same God can deal with any media magnet or political junkie. For He created all things and by Him they exist. They are all under His control, and only allowed to exist as He wills!

And just as the stubbornness of Pharaoh cost him his life, so today, the powers that be, should be careful of their actions against the people of God.

There are some of the descriptions of stubbornness, or narrowminded persons.

"A stubborn person is not willing to change their ideas or

even consider anyone-else's opinion or reason. He is not interested in ideas that are different from his own. He is opinionated, dominating, and unreasonable, very rigid, and not willing to accept that he could possibly be mistaken, or even wrong, in his opinions." (This type can also be called a Perfectionist.)

Like Pharaoh of old, he had a very high opinion of himself!

So, in the eyes of a, "brain-washed, and controlled people," Pharaoh was seen as a god!

The only problem with being "a god" is, there is no one to blame when things fall apart!

The biggest problem with being "the captain of your own ship" is, when the storms come, and come they will, you are on your own.

I preached a sermon, some years ago, entitled "What do you do when you are out, on the sea of life, and a storm arises, you are too far out to turn back, and try as you may you are making no headway." So, do you abandon ship, or do you face your storms and win!?

The idea is to keep facing the storm. Don't turn to the right or to the left. Like those disciples on the sea of Galilee, in the dark night, Keep-on-keeping-on!

Your rescuer is on His way, His name is Jesus, and He will come to you, just as He promised. So call on Him!

Along with Pharoah, *Jonah was the second, most stubborn man, in history.* He knew what to do, but he did the exact opposite.

God told him to go to Nineveh, which was inland, but Jonah rose-up and fled to Joppa, jumped on a ship and sailed toward Tarshish. He thought he could hide from God.

We all have a "personal stubborn streak toward God" and unless we surrender to Him, we will suffer the same punishment as Pharoah and Jonah.

12
Self-Measurement & Harassment

A few Sundays ago, our Pastor spoke on "The road to Revival" and these are a few of the things he said;

"We need to be measured with God's measurements.

"God measures us by our vision and our passion for that vision."

And he also said, there are _three people_ living inside of us:

1. The one we think we are.

2. The one other folks think we are.

3. And, the one God knows we are.

The apostle Paul says, "Measuring ourselves by ourselves is not wise!"

It seems that no matter how your measurements come out, there will always be someone waiting in the wings, to try to change you with their sliding rule.

And when they can't, _after a long series of phone calls and listening to the infamous recorded messages,_ "All of our professionals are busy assisting other callers. Please hold", and after ninety-nine times of hearing that recording, you hang up in despair. You know you've run into another Black-Hole called "Harassment"!

This is one of Satan's greatest, and most used, means of bringing you down to his level!

We call these midnight-crawlers "spam artists" but how

many times a day do we get another type of call; "Hello, I'm calling about your vehicle warranty, or your credit card balance, or about buying your house." At the end of the day just as you are falling off to sleep, you get this call, supposedly, from the Social Security Administration, "your social security number is being used for fraudulent purposes. Please call us immediately." You hang up and ask yourself, "who are these people?"

You, my friend, are being Harassed, whether it's by phone or by mail.

Harassment is associated with an increased risk of Anxiety, Depression, and Post-Traumatic-Stress-Disorder, also known as, PTSD, which can easily produce, a diminished capacity of self-esteem and psychological well-being.

So, how do you deal with this unseen enemy?

If you are suffering with any of these traumas in your life, don't coddle them by making excuses for them.

Begin by keeping a record of the calls and the letters, keeping records of dates, times, and conversation.

And remember that you are not alone, millions of others are dealing with the same, or different types. I have just, while typing this document, had to deal with Mr.___ from Card Services, he was so kind, all he wanted to do was lower my interest rate...???

Talk to someone about your situation.

Letting go and forgiving will help you to have some peace of mind.

Sadly though, the truth of the matter is, there are many seniors who are the target of these scam-artists, many of whom fall prey, to their ungodly schemes.

There is also a Spiritual aspect to this situation. Satan, the accuser, and liar will try anything within his power to destroy your credibility.

But you can rebuke him "in the name of Jesus" and you will find out that God is greater than these "snakes-in-the-grass, tools of evil!"

13
In Control

Recently, a friend and I were out playing golf on a windy and not so clear morning. We were always in a hot competition when it came to golf and this morning, as we approached the seventeenth hole we were in a tied game.

The next two holes would determine who would be the champ for that day. My friend, of long-standing, addressed the ball with, "And now for the coup-de-grace'" You are about to become a loser my friend, because I am about to put you out of your misery by pulling away from you for the win!

How the game turned out is not of importance here accept to say that he was wrong. But what is important is, that this is another "Black-Hole" for many of us competitive folk. It is called "The Black-Hole of CONTROL"!

We who, "have-to-always-be-in-control," can easily be sucked into that Black-Hole of despair if things don't go our way.

Isn't it ironic and even a shame, the two very close friends, cannot remain friends, simply because one of them has this diabolical need, to always be in control?!

This spirit has separated, families, friends, lovers and even "Christian brothers and sisters. So, listen-up my friend, to "always be in control" can only be attributed to God, for He's the only one with that capacity!

So, you say, "I've got it right here in my head," but listen, you need to get it into your heart. ONLY GOD has the ability to always be in control!

For all you "control freaks" this "Black-Hole" is open! And quietly whispering, "Come-into-my-parlor," says this Black-Hole to the perfectionist. You are always right, And I will help you to be "always-right."

How many relationships have been shipwrecked, by the perfectionist, in control, spirit that pervades our lives? The number is yet to be calculated.

In 1st Kings 22: it tells us of Ahab, the king of Israel who wanted to always be in control, because he wanted what he wanted, in his time, and in his way.

He was a control freak.

He not only wanted things to go his way, but he told the prophets what to prophesy. The fact is, he did not like the true prophet of God Micaiah, because he wouldn't go along with his ill-conceived plans.

Ahab even sent his hench-men to convince Micaiah that, "Everyone else is telling the King good news, so you should do the same."

But then, because Ahab was going to do what he wanted to do anyway, a lying spirit came to Ahab and said, "It's ok, go ahead with your plans."

It cost Ahab his life.

There have been many Ahab's since, and there have been many lives lost, because of that same spirit.

14
The Night Stalker

There are times when we are disturbed, in the middle of a good night's sleep, by thoughts of our past inequities. Even though these things are forgiven, try as we may, *we cannot seem to conquer those "Night-Stalkers! But we cannot let our past destroy our future!*

YESTERDAY IS GONE, TOMORROW MAY NEVER COME, WE HAVE TO LIVE FOR TODAY!

In Psalm 24:7-10 it states: "Lift up your heads, oh you gates, and be lifted up, you ancient doors, that the King of glory may come in. Who is this King of glory? The Lord strong and mighty, the Lord mighty in battle.

Lift up your heads, oh you gates; lift them up, you ancient doors, that the King of glory may come in. Who is He, this King of glory?

The Lord God Almighty—He is the King of glory."

The Apostle Paul wrote in Romans 8: 31-39 "What, then, shall we say in response to these things? If God is for us, who can be against us? He who did not spare his own Son, but gave him up for us all—how will he not also, along with him, graciously give us all things? Who will bring any charge against those whom God has chosen? It is God who justifies us. Who then is the one who condemns? No one. Christ Jesus died for us, and more than that, He was raised to life—and is at the right hand of God—and is also interceding there for us. Who shall separate us from the love of Christ? Shall trouble or hardship or persecution or famine or nakedness or danger or sword? As It is written: "For your sake we face death all day long. We are considered as sheep to be slaughtered." No, in all these things, we are more than conquerors through him who loved us. For I am convinced that neither death nor life, neither angels nor demons, neither the present nor the future, nor any powers, neither height nor depth, nor anything else in all creation, will be able to separate us from the love of God that is in Christ Jesus our Lord."

And in Romans 8:1-4, "There is therefore now, no condemnation for those who are in Christ Jesus, because through Christ Jesus the law of the Spirit who gives life has set us free from the law of sin and death.

For what the law was powerless to do because it was weakened by the flesh, God did by sending His own Son in the likeness of sinful flesh to be a sin offering for us. And so He condemned sin in the flesh, in order that the righteous requirement of the law might be fully met in us, who do not live according to the flesh but according to the Spirit."

So then, let us not be sucked-in by the Black holes of life that stalk in the darkness. That is ever looking to make us conform to their vision, and not God's vision, for us!

I was just reading the last chapters of 2nd Chronicles and the story of <u>King Josiah</u>, a great man of God. He did what was right in the sight of the Lord, and even though he had a failure at times, yet he repented, and God restored him!

But shortly after, his death the people of Israel turned against God and went back to the ways of rebellion.

I immediately wanted to go and read the book of Daniel. This is where the results are spelled out.

The choicest of Israel's young men were taken prisoners

by king Nebuchadnezzar to be restrained in his national ways.

Daniel 1:4-5 "Children in whom there was no blemish, but well favored, and skillful in all wisdom, and cunning in knowledge, and understanding science, and such as had ability in them to stand in the king's palace, and whom they might teach the learning and the tongue of the Chaldeans. And the king appointed them a daily provision of the king's meat, and of the wine which he drank: so nourishing them three years, that at the end thereof they might stand before the king."

Had they continued to serve God under the leadership of king Josiah they would not have been captured and made prisoners, but they didn't listen.

I am burdened with the needs of our country. We desperately need to repent and turn back to God. There needs to be a clarion cry to God, *"Please help us to return to the Lord God of our fathers."*

It seems that every time Israel sinned AND they turned back to God, He always restored them back to their place of FAVOR with God and peace with their enemies! Have you noticed that life tends to repeat itself and we are there again.

The "Black holes of life" have sucked many into its parlor and they are suffering the consequences.

And as the proponents of "toxic sewage" keep pumping their filth into America's lifelines, our homes, schools, and even our churches, the "politically correct" system of politics continues to sign away all our freedoms. Are we going to continue on our, as usual, "do nothing attitude?"- or will we stop the *downward sucking slide,* in our beloved country, *into the Black-Hole of insanity,* by seeking the Face of God?

We should be like Joshua of old, when he stated, *"As for ME and MY HOUSE, we will serve the Lord!"*

May we follow the actions of Joshua and King Josiah and repent, that we might see a restoration of the graciousness and beauty of our beloved country.

15
Pride Goes Before a Fall

One of the most insidious and dangerous of the Black holes is, _PRIDE._

Proverbs 8:13 God says; _"I hate pride and arrogancy"_!

Proverbs 16:18 says; _"Pride goes before destruction, and a haughty spirit before a fall."_!

The are so many brands of pride; there's Individual, Family, National, and perhaps a few more.

These have cost more and demanded more than any area of individual concern.

The Wiktionary dictionary describes Pride as "A feeling of deep satisfaction and pleasure derived from one's own achievements, from the perceived quality and value of their possessions."

This is also linked to "The perceived value of one's OWN abilities."

This is what cost Lucifer, the Archangel of Heaven who was became known as SATAN!

Jesus said; "I saw Satan fall like a stroke of lightening from Heaven."!

He had everything and Pride cost him everything!

Isaiah records in chapter 14:12-17; "How you have fallen from heaven, O morning star, son of the morning! But now you have been cast down to the earth,

You, who once laid low the nations! You said in your heart,

"I will ascend to the heavens; I will raise my throne above the stars of God;

I will sit enthroned on the mount of assembly, on the utmost heights of Mount of the congregation in the sides of the north.

I will ascend above the tops of the clouds; I will make myself like the Most High."

But you are brought down to the realm of the dead, to the depths of the pit.

NOW, those who see you stare at you, and ponder your fate: and they ask, *"is this the man who shook the earth and made the kingdoms tremble, the man who made the world a wilderness, who overthrew its cities and would not let it's captives go free?"*

This is the story of PRIDE and what it does to those who entertain it, or should we say "are infected by it"!

We also see in the book of Esther, "A man named Haman, who became prideful, after he was promoted by the King. He became a very prideful man. He became fascinated with himself! He loved the worship of others as they bowed to him when he walked by.

But Mordecai, a very religious Jew, would not bow to him! You see he believed that the GOD he served, was the only one worthy of obeisance.

But Haman became so obsessed with himself that he conned the King into signing a decree to destroy all the Jewish race.

What this prideful man did not realize was, the joke was on him!

"The Queen was also a Jew," was also Mordecai's adopted daughter.

Pride is so blinding and debilitating that you cannot see

the forest for the trees.

Under the cruel hand of this spirit, *all that matters is the big "I"* and in the end, this will lead to destruction! This Black-Hole can, and has sucked in, so many good, well-meaning folk.

Now there is still the possibility of deliverance from pride.

If we follow the advice of God's Word, then we will be victorious!

In Psalm 37:3 David says; "Trust in the Lord with all your heart and do not lean on your OWN understanding, He also says in verse, If 'In ALL your ways you acknowledge HIM, HE will direct your paths"!

'Commit your way to the Lord and He will bring your desires to completion!

In Psalm 24: 7 it says, "Lift up your heads...and let the King of Glory come in. Who is this King of Glory? "The Lord God Almighty, He is the King of Glory"!

David also prayed, "Let not mine enemies triumph over me"!

So, let's conquer that spirit of pride, because it is an enemy! and stay away from *that enemy's* powerful Sucking Black Hole.

Here's some Great advice for conquering the "spirit of Pride"!

And Pride is a spirit that *"If you don't conquer it, IT WILL CONQUER YOU"*!

It has been my experience from time and time again, to see these things in operation in the lives of many!

And please keep this in mind, as the Prophet Isaiah, in chapter 40: 10-31 says; "Look, *the Sovereign Lord who comes with power,* and rules with a mighty arm.

See, His reward is with Him, and His recompense accompanies Him.

He tends his flock like a shepherd: He gathers the lambs in His arms and carries them close to His heart; He gently leads those that *are with young.*

Who has measured the waters in the hollow of His hand, and with the breadth of His hand marked off the heavens? He has held the dust of the earth in a basket and weighs the mountains and the hills in a balance.

WHO can fathom the Spirit of the Lord, or WHO can instruct the Lord and be His counselor?

Whom did the Lord consult to enlighten Him, and who taught Him judgment, and who gave Him the knowledge, and taught Him the right way?

The nations are like a drop in a bucket; they are regarded as dust on the scales; He weighs the islands as though they were fine dust.

Before Him all the nations are as nothing; they are regarded by Him as worthless and less than nothing.

With whom, then, will you compare God?

To what image will you liken Him? HE certainly IS NOT AN Idol! Because, an idol, which is made by a metalworker, and a goldsmith are overlayed with gold and fashions of silver chains.

Do you not know? Have you not heard? Has it not been told you from the beginning? Have you not understood how the earth was formed?

GOD stretched out the heavens like a canopy and spreads them out like a tent.

He brings princes to nothing and reduces the rulers of this world to the same.

"To whom then will you compare Me, saith The Lord, or who is My equal?" says the Holy One. heavens Lift-up your eyes and look to the Heavens: Who created all these? AND who brings out the starry host one by one and calls forth each of them by name.

So why do you say, "My way is hidden from the Lord; my cause is disregarded by my God?"

Do you not know? Have you not heard? The Lord is the everlasting God, the Creator of the ends of the earth. He will not grow tired or weary, and His understanding no one can fathom.

He gives strength to the weary and increases the power of the weak.

Even youths grow tired and weary, and young men stumble and fall;

but those who hope in the Lord will renew their strength. They will soar on wings like eagles; they will run and not grow weary, they will walk and not faint.

The key to the whole matter is; Believe Gods Word to be safe - trust it to be holy - and rely on it - to avoid all those black holes and He is the answer to all your Spiritual needs.

If these "black holes of life" have sucked you into its parlor and you feel that you are about to reap their consequences, then there is one thing you need to do: *Trust in The Lord with all your heart and do not try to figure Him out!*

The solution is still a good-ol' dose of "calling-upon-The-Lord"!

The only question that remains is, what will we do?

The answer should be like Joshua of old, when he said, "As for ME and MY HOUSE, we will serve the Lord!"

AND, may we follow the actions of King Josiah, who turned the hearts of his people from Idolatrous worship AND lead them back to their True-God!

It is expedient for us to do the same in our day, so that we might see a restoration of the graciousness and beauty of our beloved country and its people.

There are those who are burning flags, tearing down

statues, destroying the unity of our great land with racial innuendos and ignoring the history that made America a great nation, all for "their-point-of-view!"

This is not a political statement –

BUT WE NEED TO TURN BACK TO GOD!!

This has always been the right thing to do and it IS still the answer to all our needs!

16
The key Ingredient

There are some important choices that must be made, and they are "a must" if we are to be victorious over these insidious black holes.

Our dependance upon the government is not a sufficient answer to it all.

With all the fear in our world, we are stressed-out beyond measure. The most sort after word in the search-mode of today's inquiries, *is FEAR*, and the most exclusive answers are unsatisfactory.

With the onslaught of the pandemic and now the world rocked by war, we are pressed beyond measure!

Lack of hope is a daily consensus from the While House to the "border dweller" under the bridge in Los Angeles, California.

So, the Blame-Game is the top story on the news and the excuses are being heard from Liberal to conservative to religious households.

We are the "stressed-out generation" who "knows-it-all" and still we seem to be unable to do anything.

Our pride is what is killing us! It is a "night-stalker" and as a result of it, fear has invaded the most cherished institutions of our day… and we are all looking for someone to blame.

The black holes are there.

They always have been and will continue to be there, so long as there is life in those bones!

The best advice is still that of Marlin my pilot, *"Bank-her-to-the-right"*!

17
The Need: UNITY

Unity of purpose is a great need in all our lives!

Some years ago, I was driving thru down-town Nassau and was amazed by the traffic jams and the torn-up streets. So I asked a policeman who was just standing there, just as amazed as I was. "Sir, why is the traffic so snarled & unorganized?" His statement to me was astounding, "Sir", he said, "it's because our utility companies are afraid to trust each other." When one digs to bury a cable, the other is not notified. As soon as the electrical company repaired the roads from their digs, the phone company comes along and digs-up the same roads for their cables. So there's always *holes in the roads*, thus all the traffic, jams, as you can see!"

I remembered that *The Nassau Guardian*, the local newspaper, had a front page headline entitled, "Why all the snarls in our streets?"

I thought back at the 911 fiasco in New York city, when all of our agencies, the FBI, the CIA, Homeland security etc., - were so suspicious of each other that they would not share "their intelligence" between each other, thus we had the "Twin-Towers-Disaster. The whole country suffered, and the President was blamed!

Too often we blame each other, and even God, for disasters that could've been avoided had we sought help and co-operated with each other.

Someone wrote this; "If you put 100 *black ants* and 100 *red ants* in a jar, nothing will happen.

But if you shake the jar hard enough, the ants will attack and kill each other.

The red ants will consider the *black ants* to be *their enemies* and so will the black ants consider the red ants to be *their enemies.*

But the real enemy is the one who shook the jar!

The same thing is happening in our society.

So before we attack each other, we should stop and think about who's shaking the jar!

This scenario has been going on from the beginning, Adam blamed Eve, Eve blamed the serpent and *the serpent who is the shaker of the jar) blamed God.* Thus the whole world is suffering under the curse of sin!

Dr. Richard Dobbins said; "Sin is an invisible force, that emanates from Satan and it impacts the *mind* to stimulate the *brain* to *think* in terms of *life choices which distract from and destroys one's Divine potential"*

The same is so with the lack of unity. *The disunity of our efforts* has separated us and set our country on the road to disaster, from under the bridge in Los Angeles to the harbor in New York City.

But there is a solution to this dilemma- *it is found in the words of the Psalmist (#133:)..* "Behold, how good and how pleasant it is for brethren to dwell together in unity! It is like precious ointment poured upon the head, that runs down upon the beard, even Aaron's beard: that went down to the skirts of his garments;

It is like the dew of Hermon, and as the dew that descended upon the mountains of Zion: *for there the LORD commanded His blessing, even life for evermore."*

At the time of the writing of this Psalm Israel was under the leadership of Judges. They were under One-Common-Leader.

They would march together to Jerusalem for worship and this Psalm was written as a marching tune for the trek. The people sang as they walked. It helped them not to notice the rough roads and to put all their energies into reaching their goal.

It called for "harmony," *a musical term meaning "The* absence of discord *and* a pleasing sound." It is "A dwelling together" – to dwell AS ONE! -- this -)(- Hebrew letter gives us the meaning of *"even-together"* It carries the tenor of *"being at a live concert".*

I remember my daughter and I attended a Dallas Holm concert in West Palm Beach, we bought a tape of the concert and played it on the way home - My daughter remarked, "The music takes on a different sound from what we heard at the concert".

You see, we had something to measure by and that's what made the difference.

This is what Unity does, it helps everything, all our efforts, to work better!

The only way to conquer those "Black holes" that pop-up and try to direct and even destroy our lives, is to turn those curses into blessings!

Here are a few illustrations that may help:
(1). Two tough ol' mules, tied together, said,

Get this you dope:
We're tied together with the same rope,
The one was constantly saying to the other
You come my way and I'll get a nibble of that bale of hay-
I won't said the other, you come my way!
I want some of that hay don't you see.
So, they got nowhere, they dug into the ground.
All they did was pull each other down.
Then they turned about, those stubborn mules and said,
We're acting just like those human fools...
Why not let's pull together and we'll both get hay?
So they ate some hay and they even liked it too.
They said let's be friends good and true
And as the sun went down, they were heard to say,
Ahhhh, this is the end of a perfect day!

(2). During a Sunday morning service, the pastor noticed a visitor come into the church and march right down to the front row and sit down.

Shocked, the pastor went to the visitor after the service and asked, "How is it that you being a visitor came right down to the front row to sit"? "Sir, I'm a bus driven", said the man, "I just came to see how you could get all these people to sit in the rear of the building?"

Sometimes we all would like to run away from our problems.

Here's two more illustrations that might help.

(3). "I'm running away from home" said seven year old Linda, who had a suitcase in her hand, heading out the door. In obvious surprise her dad did not try to stop her or even talk her out of it.

He only reminded her that she was always welcome to

return home anytime she pleased. There was no reasoning as to why she was running away, but the dad called the neighbor down the road and asked them to lookout for her as she passed by.

The neighbor informed him that she was already at their house with no apparent reason for being there. Later in the afternoon the dad called again and inquired as to her situation, asking the neighbor to let her know that he hoped she'd be home in time for dinner, which was very soon.

She came home running and crying and we held her close. In a few minutes she calmed down and in a burst of pseudosophistication she quipped, "That was a nice place to visit, but I wouldn't want to live there." *She never ran away from home again*!

A good example of our Heavenly Father, toward prodigals, who run away from Home!

(4). I love this analogy:
When God created fish, He spoke to the sea.
When God created trees, He spoke to the earth.
But when God wanted to create MAN, He turned to Himself and said, "Let Us make man in Our image and Our likeness!

Here's something to consider:
If you take a fish out of water, it dies!
If you remove a tree from the soil it dies!
Likewise, when MAN is disconnected from GOD, he dies!
God is man's natural environment. We were created to live in His presence!

We must be *connected to Him* because it is only *in Him* that LIFE exists!

Water without fish is still just water- but a fish without water is dead.

Soil without a tree is just soil, but a tree without soil is dead!

God without man is still GOD, - But man without God is nothing –

So let's stay connected to God!

There is a good lesson taught us in 2nd Chronicles 30:7-9 "And be not you like your fathers, and like your brethren, which trespassed against the LORD God of their fathers, who gave them up to the desolation, as ye see.

Now, don't you be stiff-necked, as your fathers were, but yield yourselves unto the LORD, and enter His sanctuary, which He hath sanctified forever: *and serve the LORD your God, that the fierceness of His wrath may turn away from you.*

For if you turn again unto the LORD, your brethren and your children shall find compassion before them that lead them captive, *so that they shall come again into this land:* for the LORD your God is gracious and merciful, and will not turn away His face from you, *if you return unto Him.*"

18
It Takes *a Daily Commitment*

We live in a world of INSTANTS; *everything has to be done* NOW!

But in reality, it does not work that way!

Only God can have perfect timing, and He will never give-up control to *imperfect humans*, who want, what they want, *and want IT NOW*! Many "a break-thru" has been delayed, for many years, because God knows *more than you or me*.

There is a few verses in Isaiah's writings chapter 43:2.

"When you pass through the waters, I will be with you; *and when* you pass through the rivers, *they will not sweep over you. When you walk* through *the fire*, you will not be burned; the flames will not set you ablaze. For I am the LORD your God!"

NOW, He does not say "IF you" BUT "WHEN YOU"!!

The word "*WHEN*" means "you had better be prepared!"

So in order to be in a race:

First. You must ENTER!

Second. You must SHOW-UP!

Third. You must be ON TIME!

No stopping at Dunkin Donuts for coffee!

Remember God sets the TIME for the race to begin and end!

Fourth. You must Stay focused!

You must decide what your goal is - and you must decide what your plan is to reach that goal!

Remember, A horse gets nowhere until he is harnessed! And you will not be delivered unless you respond to God!

Also remember "Your enemy is looking to stop you at every turn"!

It will take a *"Daily commitment"* to win *and* God wants you to be victorious!

Hebrews 12:1-2; "we are surrounded by such a great cloud of witnesses, so let us throw off everything that hinders us and the sin that so easily entangles us. And let us run with perseverance the race marked out for us, fixing our eyes on Jesus, the pioneer and perfecter of our Faith!"

It will take a REAL Commitment, on our part, to avoid those Black Holes along the way and continue to be committed to the task before us!

Sometimes, the things that hinder us the most can be our best victory, that is "If we can see beyond the moment".

We assumed that the Pandemic was a disaster, But there are at least SIX things that we learned from that unholy distraction;

1. It changed our priorities!

2. We learned how to love people that we didn't even know!

3. We learned how to respond to our assignments!

4.. Even though people may have thought that we were Supermen, we learned how to "Take-off-our-capes"!

5. We learned that it was OUR responsibility to fulfill OUR OWN assignments!

6. We learned how to avoid Bitterness, Bigotry, & Bondage, "How to keep our car running by stopping more often at the gas station!"

We also learned that those who spread HATE, will be the

recipients of hate themselves!

Remember this, "When others may see *A SHEPHERD BOY, GOD* may see *A KING!*"

We need to look inside more often – the Pandemic drove us to that and more!

For all you church goers who are disillusioned with the way things have gone in your season, someone wrote this:

"If you're looking for the kind of church, like the kind of church *you like,*

You needn't pack your grip and take a long, long trip,

Cause you'll only find what you've *left behind,* that it's not the church, IT'S YOU!"

Come on all you warriors, fight the good fight and win - over all those black holes, that pop-up in your space!!

A Companion Study Guide
How to Face Life's Black Holes and Overcome

A Brief Message to the Teacher
(before each session)

Before the lesson that you are about to teach, take a special time each day, to pray for your class and also pray over the lesson that you are about to teach, so as to ensure that the group will comprehend what you are sharing with them.

Depending on the date, the time and place of your study, you could prepare some refreshments for before or after the lesson time.

Prepare and hand out an advance copy of, the discussion questions, you will be looking into for that session, so that the class can be well prepared.

Always open and close with prayer!

If questions come up that you cannot answer at the time, be honest and ask for some time to research the answer...Be genuine!

God will give you the wisdom to give an appropriate answer to every question.

Introduction

This is a companion to the book, "How to Face Life's Black Holes _and Overcome._" And it is written to help those who are struggling to survive through the pandemic-C19 and all that followed, including the war waging on Ukraine, and all the price changes that are taking place in our stress upon stress world!

The goal of the author is to endeavor to bring about some semblance of grace and peace, into the lives of those who are hurting the most, from these "Signs of the times," - these horrific days that we are living in.

Our nation, and the world, is in a time of political unrest _like has never been known._ This is the beginning of the fulfillment of the prophesies of Jesus and the Apostle Paul when they said; "In the last days perilous times will come," which we are seeing come to pass, _and hopefully they will pass._

May God bless you as you study and try to be as honest as possible, to give a reasonable answer, to some of the questions of the students.

It is my hope that you, and your students, may be at peace in a world where there is no peace, and - as Moses wrote in Numbers 6:22-27, "MAY The LORD bless you, and keep you: The LORD make His face shine upon you, and be gracious unto you: An may The LORD lift His countenance upon you and give you peace."

And as Jesus said in John 14:27, "Peace I leave with you MY PEACE I give unto You,

"*Not as the world gives, do I give to you, so don't let your hearts be troubled!*"

Black Holes questions

Chapter 1

1. What are some of the black holes that tempt you?

2. To whom can you go to get real help?

3. To start with, how can you avoid the black hole of temptation?

Chapter 2

1. What is the basis for a panic-attack?

2. How can you counteract your fears?

Chapter 3

1. When a decision MUST be made, what are some of the things you can rely on to make sure that it is the right one?

Chapter 4

1. What do you do to face some of your fears and overcome them?

2. What scripture verses have been helpful in your time of panic or fear?

Chapter 5

1. Where should we look for help when we feel lost and hopeless?

2. How can, assuming guilt for something, damage our lives?

Chapter 6

1. How can we avoid "stinkin-thinkin"?

2. What kind of life should we strive to live?

Chapter 7

1. What are some of the *things worth knowing,* in life?

2. Can improving your health also improve your cognitive skills?

Chapter 8

1. How can you differentiate between excuses and legitimate reasons?

2. What are some scriptures that might strengthen you when you face Satan's barbs?

Chapter 9

1. What steps can you take to deal with stress in your life?

2. Does stress attack only certain kinds of people?

Chapter 10

1. What are some of the dangers of "Psychic-services"?

2. Who is the only one who can *know and determine* the future?

Chapter 11

1. What are some of the pitfalls of stubbornness?

2. How can we overcome stubbornness in our lives?

Chapter 12
1. Who are the three people living inside us?

2. What are some of the things harassment can bring on a person?

Chapter 13
1. What are some dangers of always having to be in control?

2. How can we allow God to be the one in control?

Chapter 14
1. What scriptures can you use to deter the "Night Stalker?:

2. Can we do anything about the "toxic sewage" that comes into our homes?

Chapter 15
1. What are some of the dangers of pride?

2. What scriptures verse(s) will help you overcome the black hole of pride?

Chapter 16

1. How can we combat lack of hope in our lives?

2. How can you "bank her to the right" in what you are facing?

Chapter 17

1. What is the meaning of harmony and how does it apply to our lives.

2. How can we let our life choices distract us from our divine potential?

Chapter 18

1. What is your game plan for a daily commitment?

2. What might be some things that will hinder you from achieving complete victory in the area of commitment?

About the Author

Courtney Harding was born on Long Island in the southern Bahamas. At the age of twelve years, with his father's blessing, he worked with a construction crew on another island. He also worked on several ships as a chef until settling in Nassau where he was introduced to and accepted Christ as his Savior.

Courtney attended North Central University in Minneapolis, Minnesota where he earned a Bachelor of Arts degree in Bible and Pastoral Theology. He built churches in Ohio, Florida and in the Bahamas.

He presently resides in Lakeland, Florida where he recently retired from being on staff at Southeastern University.